Radiation Diary
Return to the Sea

Radiation Diary
Return to the Sea

Walter Bargen

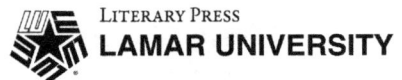
Literary Press
LAMAR UNIVERSITY

Copyright © 2023 by Walter Bargen
All rights reserved

ISBN: 978-0-9915321-9-3
Library of Congress Control Number: 2023945604

Author photo credit: Bill Palmer

Lamar University Literary Press
Beaumont, Texas

ACKNOWLEDGMENTS

I would like to express my appreciation for all who partake of the Reflection Critique group, for their reading of early versions of these poems and sharing their insights, their wit, and their wisdom: Matt Dube, Sharon Feltman, Lynne Jenkins-Lampe, Barbara Leonard, Lois Long, Zak Wardell, and Cami Wheir.

OTHER BOOKS BY WALTER BARGEN

At the Dead Center of Day
The Body of Water
Days Like This Are Necessary: New & Selected Poems
Endearing Ruins (Liebenswerte Ruinen)
The Feast
Fields of Thenar
Gone West (Ganz im Westen)
Harmonic Balance
My Other Mother's Red Mercedes
Mysteries in the Public Domain
Perishable Kingdoms
Pole Dancing in the Night Club of God
Quixotic
Remedies for Vertigo
Rising Waters
Theban Traffic
Three-Corner Catch
Too Late to Turn Back
Too Quick for the Living
Trouble Behind Glass Doors
Until Next Time
Vertical River
Water Breathing Air
West of West
Yet Other Waters
You Wounded Miracle

I want to thank the editors of the following magazines who were kind enough to select these poems to appear in their pages:

13 Miles from Cleveland	"Late, Later, Latest"
Alien Buddha Zine	"Ashes"
Concho River Review	"Beyond Beyond"
Dragon Poets Review	"Headstone"
Lothlorien Poetry Journal	"Little League"
	"Return to the Sea"
	"Ultima Thule"
Moon City Review	"After the Operation"
San Pedro River Review	"Friday at Volunteer Park"
Sow's Ear	"Radiated"
Today's Farmer	"Misdiagnosed Eclipse"
Until Next Time	"Washed Up"

Table of Contents

~ Ending the Beginning ~

1	Beyond Beyond
2	After the Operation
3	Radiated

~ Return to the Sea ~

7	Day 1	Custom Duties
9	2	Tattoo of Days
10	3	Conestoga
12	4	Late, Later, Latest
14	5	Arabic to English to German
15	6	2,000 Light Years from Home
17	7	Underemployed
18	8	Hands of the Linear Accelerator
20	9	Cracking the Code
22	10	Along the Trail
24	11	Headstone
26	12	Shadow Bands
28	13	Center Piece
29	14	Friday at Volunteer Park
31	15	Misdiagnosed Eclipse
33	16	Any Week Now
35	17	Populus Deltoides or Pinus Echinata?
37	18	Revelry
40	19	Table Dates
42	20	Camaraderie
43	21	Sea Space in the Parking Lot
44	22	Revolution Number Nine
46	23	Treading Time
47	24	Seven Miscalculations
49	25	RSVP/RIP
51	26	Sunday
52	27	Six Left

54	28 Ultima Thule
55	29 Little League
57	30 Row, Row, Row Your Dream
59	31 The Sea Shall Free Us
60	32 Decompression
61	33 Caught in the Undertow
62	34 Four Minutes and Thirty-Three Seconds
63	35 Washed Up
64	36 Return to the Sea
65	37 Ashes
66	38 At Five in the Afternoon

~End Over End~

69	39 Body Heist
70	40 Why Twenty-Two Equals Thirty-Eight Divided by Seven

Some people love death so much
they want to give it to everyone.
Dana Levin

Death was singing in the shower.
Death was happy to be alive.
Tom Robbins

Watching the pier as the ship sails away . . .
Mark Strand

~ Ending the Beginning ~

Beyond Beyond

No matter what I do, no matter how much I forget
about what I've done, no matter how much I forget
what I'm doing, no matter if I come up
with all the wrong reasons, I wander out of sight
without comrades or luggage. With wrong right
and right wrong, I learn to travel light, but never with speed
enough to escape the gravity of days and decades, winning
and losing different corners in the same dank cell.

I won't come back from this wounded earth,
raw and erased quickly by spindly weeds, no matter
how many claims I leave behind, with or without
the trail of Gretel's crumpled Post-it notes, there never was
any choice. Yes, a will to be free but not free will.
It's in the timing and yet little to do with the ticking
or flashing of watches, this measured context that contains me,
schedules me, even as the door slams behind and over me.

More or less, too much. My urgent calculations
blindly guide and obstruct every step of the way
even in my desperation to step away. Clinging to a promise,
resolution is not transformation much less disappearance,
as my soul is polished into a bright darkness,
as others see the backs of my head in the airport concourse,
or they stand on the terminal sidewalk waiting for the light
to change and shouting out my name that I no longer remember.

After the Operation

everyone wants to know,
when I meet them on street corners,
on the broken backs of sidewalks,
at a benchless pocket park
where everyone wears a trench coat;
and if I meet them in a pictureless hallway,
in an elevator headed for the 13th floor,
at the water fountain where the Ark surfs bubbles
looking for landfall as the glass fills,
in the breakroom decorated with paper banners:
wishing us more birthdays, years of anniversaries,
flowered fields of retirement, in the closet
but don't tell, in offices with doors
opened and closed, again don't tell;
at the airport waiting in line to check in,
waiting in line to be checked out:
felt up, wanded, x-rayed—only to wait in line
to board, wait in line to be seated,
greeted, offered water, coffee, soda,
and a small packet of too-salty pretzels,
as we buckle ourselves in awkward seats,
ready or not to transcend all that we know,
and everyone wants to know anyway and I say
getting along, getting by, and just maybe getting down.

Radiated

We are all hope and desperate for certainty.
Believing to know is better than not knowing,
That there is room for planning and planning means
Control and foresight, then spending
The rest of our lives running from any such scheme,
That is to know is to know too much,
That the destruction of beliefs and deconstruction of deceptions
Will outlive us but even then we have our doubts.
To keep us warm, whether running fast is enough
Or running at all will alter the end, or turning to face
What's coming, but not the other cheek,
Even that gesture is too late,
Though an elegant flourish might be remembered fondly,
Bravely, but the coming, the going indistinguishable.
Impossible to know where and when the turn
Is made, a doppelganger talking to itself,
And when Wilhelm Röentgen's wife, Anna Bertha
Ludwig, declared, "I have seen my death,"
It was enough and not enough
To see and to know, or better not to know in the seeing.
This light that did not behave like any known light
As though any light was a spotlight on the living,
Then the living dead, then the dead living, then the cold
That she felt even as the skin on the back of her hands
Reddened, lesions scaled, peeled, and no way for Wilhelm,
Discoverer of the X-ray, the *Röntgenstrahlen*,
To know all the breakage to come, exposed
So clearly, and still it was breakage, the pain undeniable,
The carpal and metacarpal disjointed, the phalanges knotted,
The digits finally unaccountable for their inactions.

~ Return to the Sea ~

Day 1 Custom Duties

I keep hearing last words though I can't recall a single one.
I keep thinking this is the song that should be played
as everyone quietly sinks into their pews,
into themselves, down through their sandals
and into the floor to walk back into the world.
Then there's the next song on the CD,
and I can't decide which ditty, tune, riff,
is most delinquently memorable.
I smell bouquets of flowers though I can't
identify a single pungent scent.

It's the common complaint, too little too late
yet either way is enough.
It has to be enough. Any declaration of weights
and measures sure to come to no consequence
or conclusion. Unanimated and soulless the body weighs
the same as it passes through all the forgotten customs.

∞

Only two, rather than two dozen,
hummingbirds returned this spring.
My mind hair-triggered for apocalypse, yet another species
flying too far away to recall, along with the monarch,
half of them frozen to death this past winter in Mexico
and the other half ashes in California fires.

∞

The joke I share with nurse Amanda about picking up
some Smith & Wesson cough syrup from the pharmacy
on the way home doesn't get a laugh.

∞

I keep cutting back on the sugar water
in the feeder and still it ferments, and still
I keep replacing it for the two loyal feathered survivors.
Then late summer, when I begin my treatment,
another dozen iridescent ruby-throated flashes appear,
enough to be a scintillating mirror ball around the feeder
hanging from an oak branch in the middle of the day
in the front yard. Gone a couple of days later.

2   Tattoo of Days

Poe cornered the market on ravens and *forever more*,
but neither forever nor more of forever
survived the centuries of empty promises.
Both roost on my shoulders plucking
clumps of hair with their beaks
as the balding pages of night keep turning.

My daughter-in-law, after many arguments
with her parents, has one tattoo, a raven that reaches
from her left shoulder to just above the elbow.
I tell her that I now have more tattoos
than she does. These three she will never see.
I think I have located two of them.

Not the one on my right hip, it's lost amid freckles,
though the technicians assure me they know the location.
Tattoos the size of pin heads, though I can't begin
to count how many angels dance there
or know if there's much chance
of their surviving the radiation.

Lying on the table, the nurse parts
my pubic hair, hence, the easiest point to find.
I make the mistake—squeezing time
out of forever until I'm haunted
by the longing, at least, for awhile,
in Poe's end, in the raven's end,
in my end. I can only distract
myself for so long. It means nothing
but this body a navigation chart folded
too many times to find a way out
of all the creases.

3   Conestoga

The wagons are circling.
The attack starts each morning at 7:30
in the dealership waiting room.
I hear the pounding of hooves
on four walls of flat screens
tuned to the news: earthquakes,
and children running out of schools
to the splatter of gunshots, reruns
of reality shows, and jittery black
& white Westerns, that surround
the customers waiting for their cars,
their signatures on the repair bills of surrender.

Captured by a customer service agent,
the third car owner stares from an armchair
at a clogged cabin air filter
where mice were working on a nest.

I'm told that the rear passenger
backup bulb is burned out.
I'm the fourth car owner
in ten minutes that needs
a new air filter. The garage must
hire mice after their evictions
as part-time agents without benefits.

But everything else looks good
for the long drive north to Lake Superior.
There to sprawl on a sickle-shaped island beach
that harvests sand, sea, and stars;
where small flocks of Canada geese
are almost close enough to touch,
then beat down the surface before landing
a little farther out of reach in a little deeper water.
But that was years ago, when a universe
rushed in below the moon's full belly

and the unmoored beach fell upward.
Now to drive there in hope
of finding a life again.

In an hour, the car is ready.
The mechanic places his screwdrivers
back in the drawer, wipes his wrenches clean,
completes the computer record
of the car's service.

If only it is this easy, now that I'm not alone
driving with my body for company
though the passenger seat is empty,
headed to the next appointment.

4   Late, Later, Latest

The beginning of August, the first rush
of autumn pours blue through the window,
floods the bed. Sure to induce the bends
if I surface too quickly. A cardinal's bloody
aria knifes the air.

Of course, I'm on the edge of late,
a word often used in Botswana
for those who are more than late.
Later than ever before.
Later than they will ever be again.
We must be patient in our waiting.

I speed past the cattail-choked pond
trying to make my first appointment.
The three-decades-old station wagon
points one way as I turn
the other into Friday morning traffic.

The receptionist asks, *How am I doing?*
My answer, *I'm here*, she nods her head.

In the treatment room, I'm running with cats
though only the linear accelerator is purring.
On my back, lines of red lasers glitter
across my lower abdomen. A lead shield
positioned over my genitals. Spangled in a ticker tape
of light, I'm a half-naked parade going nowhere,
starting at 10:30 a.m., five days a week
for the next eight weeks.

The music from speakers hang high
in each corner of the treatment room.
Radar Love, Teen Angel, My Boyfriend's Back
Pours down. I feel the notes enter my pelvis
and wonder at the extent of the damage.

Back in the subwaiting room,
wrapped in a faded blue gown,
I see cattails lining the road
that's cheaply framed and painted,
hanging on the wall across from
where I sit. Late comes
for everyone and not just today.
I happen to be early,
having written down the wrong time.

5   Arabic to English to German

Too many one ways,
too many short dead-end streets—
it's a struggle to find the address
to deliver a bicycle and quilt
to a Syrian family that speaks no English.

The house fits the description.
There's an inner door and no doorbell.
Told to be loud, I drive my knuckles
into the door. I worry it sounds
like the police or a dictator's fist.
I ask if this is the Ali family.
Confusion confounds six children
too curious to ignore the stranger.

We speak Arabic to English and back
through a nearly instantaneous
phone app translator. We sit on the living room
floor, either side of a coffee table crowded
by a mountain range of second-hand overstuffed furniture.
We eat freshly baked baklava and drink cardamom-spiced
coffee. I leave with thank you, *Inshallah*, and a plate of baklava.

At lunch a friend says his great-grandfather
grew up in a small Texas town
where only German was spoken. When his family
moved into a house near Ft. Sam Houston
in the middle of WWI, his name quickly changed
and his grandfather learned English in record time.

I wonder what language my body is learning?
Radiation opens and closes, leaves me waiting
on both sides of the leaded door.
I wait for the oncologist to translate,
to diagnose a destination, an arrival time,
maps of blood and soft tissue unclear,
the doctor says 70% chance.
One day turning away, I will drive on.

6   2,000 Light Years from Home

The weekend edition still dry, still a dollar-fifty,
even after a night of rain. No one stops to buy
a copy as cold air rushes from the grocery's
sliding glass doors. Shoppers pass, avoid eye
contact, feign interest in their companions,
admire what they've gathered in their carts,
stare at phone screens, perhaps fret being late
for an appointment, but always there's a furtive
glance, curious, concerned, over the bench sitter.

My friend arrives having arranged to meet at two
in the afternoon, ahead of Lorca by three hours,
the Spanish still digging through 90-year-old mass graves
for explanations. Her husband is seventy-nine today.
I'm ten years younger and no closer to any truth
that stands up on its own out of a grave.

I give her a birthday card and small piece
of fossilized wood once marooned on a sandbar,
work of the river's polishing rush south.
She hands me a small white bag
with a card and four pairs of socks.
The card pictures Da Vinci's naked man
each of his four legs color-penciled with bright
striped socks that match the just received gift
and his own desire untouched at the center of it all.

Socks to walk the clinic's halls, I'm told.
My feet will be a storm of color
under a fading patient's pale-blue gown.
Something to draw a nurse's attention.
There were five pairs in the bag,
one for each day of the work week,
but her husband liked the pair
with red and yellow chili pepper pattern.
It's his birthday. So the fifth day

of the weekly regime, Friday, I'll wear white
cotton socks. This will be my angelic day
as I flutter into the weekend to recover.

The card that I give her, pictures an erupting
Mt. St. Helens, smoke billowing into the sky,
as if earth's engines are fired and working full speed,
steaming toward Alpha Centauri, knowing
we will never live long enough to catch up.

7   Underemployed

Up each morning at 7, it's my new job.
I thought I'd forgotten the routine,
retired, but there it is, the alarm clock beating
its silly face with the skinniest arms, suggesting
the final stages of illness, but hands larger
than a president's, who's threatening
to radiate the world.

First I feed more cats than I have fingers and toes.
There are the litter boxes to be cleaned.
Water bowls emptied and refilled.
The unhappy cats that have pills shoved
down their throats each day and cats
that are given an insulin shot twice a day.
There's delinquent raccoons who demand
their share of the dog food but there isn't a dog around,
and the foxes who peaceably compete with the raccoons.
There's the hummingbird feeders that are drained
before I wake up and need more sugar water. The bird seed
to be scattered for the usual late summer suspects.

After the shower, I don't have time for breakfast,
though I don't want to offend the technicians,
that is, I don't want to offend as my hospital gown
is opened and I lay on the table and the monstrous
machine is aligned with my dot tattoos
that surround my hips. That's my job for eight weeks,
to lie still for fifteen minutes and be penetrated.
The spotless white machine purrs around
the table dishing out a deadly living.

8   Hands of the Linear Accelerator

∞

The sweaty man who, years ago, sliced
off his finger, wears a hollow prosthesis
to conceal the vial of chicken blood.
He refuses to roll up his cuffs
and expose his forearms.
He stands before the congregation
ready to make them believe.
A sheet of butcher paper suspended
above the body clots with black spots.
The shadows of arms and legs appear.
The diagnosis and prognosis:
the Bible flung against a bare back
sticks, a sullen lump of chapters
and verses that refuse to fall to the floor.

∞

A fevered tongue speaks. The diseased
come forth, disrobe, lay their afflictions
on blanketed tables under a tropical roof
without walls. Burning moths over a burning
body, his hands flutter, hover, dive into
the searing bulge of an abdomen.

A chest pierced, fingers submerge,
blood floods the soft crevices
of a sagging geography and puddles
on the sheet. He kneads the skin squeezing
malevolence into a wooden bowl.
He opens a gash, roots, probes
draws out the festering.
He withdraws his bloody stumps
followed by his hands.
Then his fingers disappear into a forehead,
circle around the back of an eye,
return with a cadaverous slippage
left displayed on top of a bloody chest.

Other days there are accusations
of chopped cow's liver, blood too
red, too watery, or too black before
it kisses the air. But it's what he found.
The naked stand and dress without wound
or scar, without embarrassment,
without their lifelong suffering.

∞

How does one body pass into
and through another, not leaving
a stitched trail, not a single cry of pain?
There are the infinities of the subatomic,
space suspended on top of space,
where love ends and ends again in gratitude,
where hands are lost and found,
found and lost again, centuries of August
in any moment, the truth of one day
becoming truer in the moment of many days,
the visible wounds always less
than the invisible, the believers
achieving their perfections, losing
an eye or nose to a hand, before
they see again, before they breathe again.

9   Cracking the Code

∞

Once a week, I see the radiologist in his office,
as if I've been a bad boy and must confess
my transgressions. Forgot to drink a pint of water
yesterday to inflate my bladder to keep the plumbing
separated from the area to be treated. Forgot to wear
loose clothing in case my skin reddens
if the beam dances too intimately
across a patch of skin.
Its fiery pirouettes will only be worsened
by elastic bands and belts.
Forgot to say my prayers with every breath
even though each breath is its own weak prayer.

∞

There is a fungus that grows on the floor
of tropical rain forests, it waits for hard-shelled
insects to scuttle past. Eventually, the fungus burns a hole
through the exoskeleton, devours the unnecessary organs,
then the unnecessary parts of the insect's brain.
In control, it directs the creature
up the bark of a tree to the forest canopy,
sometimes a hundred feet high. At the top,
the shell splits open and the fungal
spores disperse to drift through the air
to land far from where this insecticide began.
During treatment I struggle to remember
the fungus' name. Later I find out
it could be *Ophiocordyceps unilateralis*
(Sometimes called the Zombie Ant fungus.)
or *Crytococcus neoformans*.
This is what happened to me,
the shell around the prostate cracked,
the cancer spread. Is it early enough or too late?
The fungus is the source on an anti-rejection
drug for organ transplants. Rainforests the size
of Delaware cut down and burned each week.

∞

Back in the car, I listen to escalating rhetoric
between two mad men on opposite sides
of the planet. The citizens of Guam are instructed
not to risk permanent blindness by staring
at the flash of a nuclear explosion,
as if there will be anything left to see.
After the initial detonation they are to remove
all clothing, embarrassment filed away to a past life;
to wash hair but not use a conditioner,
beauty orphaned to the next millennium;
and if nothing else is available revert to the 1950s
strategy of duck and cover. At the stoplight
on Broadway and Ninth I wonder, would
I get a cost-free treatment to end
all this if I was living on Guam?

10   Along the Trail

∞

Ok, flying seven miles above the earth,
above the horizons of street and stoplights,
houses that stretch beyond belief,
owners who grasp no more than their yards
and another night with beer and Doritos,
listening to another losing game
or watching a cheap 80s zombie fest,
if the local news hasn't filmed one live.
Once someone thought
all these buildings a good idea.

∞

I'm told, comforted, that I receive no more
radiation than during a flight to the coast
or from a dentist's quick black
& white glimpse of my bushel basket of teeth:
drilled, filled, crowned, and ready to devour the world
one small bite at a time. I'm supposed to feel better
in the reclined chair in the examination light's glare,
ready to declare my guilt as I work to overthrow
this body. I don't have a ticket to anywhere
but a carbon-fiber table.

∞

Months later, after the shock of urinating blood,
once again lying on a table
in the doctor's office,
after the cystography,
after watching the camera display
the inside image of my bladder
projected on a computer screen,
I see maybe a hundred black fish
aligned in one direction as if suspended
in a current, or a field of burned leaves
still clinging to their stalks, or flesh charred
by radiation. Is this ticket refundable?

∞

On the ceiling above the table,
not centered on my face,
closer to my feet, I imagine
where I will be walking when I leave here.
It's a back-lit 3 x 3 foot photograph on a transparent panel,
a green mountain meadow crowded with the white candles
of flowering bear grass and the blush of Indian paintbrush.
I will be looking down at the rocks and rough terrain
of each step along this trail. But when the linear accelerator
makes its move to devour me, the mountain beyond
and the flowers are obscured, shrouded in clouds and snow.
High up the slope, my destination, the empty eye-sockets
of an exposed escarpment with its ice-choked, shattered grimace.

∞

I'm thinking mimicry will save me,
if I can just get out of this glowing chrysalis
to become a viceroy protected
by the monarch butterfly's poisonous presence.
What will save the viceroys if the monarchs
fly beyond this realm? I see a photograph of thousands
of dead blackened monarchs in the Sierra Madres of Mexico
decorating the drifts of an unexpected late spring snow
not unlike what I see on the screen of the cystography.

11   Headstone

In addition to radon, naturally occurring radioactive minerals (NORMS) in granite and marble can emit small amounts of beta and gamma radiation. —EPA Report (2018)

Museum scholars decried the bust's authenticity,
a forger's rendition of an ancient past:
thick locks of marble-carved hair flow over
a youthful forehead, curls almost touch
his eyebrows, more like tongues of Vesuvian
lava than hair, more sixties rebellion
or disheveled nineteenth century Romantic flare,
the beard more muttonchops teased
into a satyr's goatee, nothing that conceals
his thin cold lips that cannot speak, and now sits
restored and mounted on a pedestal. This perfect
Roman youth would argue against
the genuine Mountains of the Moon dolomite
and cry for flesh—flesh even two millennia later.

How can we know except not one of us ready
to surrender to anything less than caress,
even walking the cemetery rows, following
the carefully selected and highly polished,
the fluted and vined, the angelic and cherubic,
the deeply incised names, the carved
portraits, the photographs, the small video
screens and audio messages tripped by
vigilant electric eyes, all embedded
in marble. The deceased cease the passerby
amid all the daily accounting and ask
is this the real one, death so unoriginal
even when it's authentic.

Two museum busts of young Pompey face each other.
One Thasian surface is not metamorphosed,
not encrusted, not microscopically rounded

by weather. This time it's the bust
with the busted nose and chipped chin,
the less than perfect one that leaves us disbelieving,
even as the unblemished marble perfects the coldest flesh.

12   Shadow Bands

Just before and just after is what I know.
Between happens too fast. I listen to the gears whirl.
The linear accelerator stalks, ungainly,
monstrous, something out of a 50s Japanese
Mothra movie, if it wasn't so laughably mechanical.

A single polished plastic egg that no one is going
to steal as it slowly rotates around the table
where I'm belly up, the ghost of a fish bobbing
on the dried up lake bed of time. It swings in
from the right with its red teeth ready to chew
on what's inside me, laying its egg to hatch later,
the bet is on much later. The doctor tells me
that something else, shark, snake, asteroid, nuclear
war, will get me first. What about climate change?

A small arm swims toward me
with no thought of rescue. I can't move.
There's no lifeguard hurtling
down the beach, hurling a surfboard
into the radiant waves; no rescue crew
dragging a dory into the turbulent surf of electrons,
paddles failing to gain purchase
over the next ripping atomic crest;
no hovering helicopter's blades backwash
flattening a small coin of radiated sea
as it lowers a cable that never reaches
the victim, and so I drown, and drown again
each day in the whirring surf of a machine
that controls the ebb and flow of fission.

Not unlike the most ephemeral shadow bands,
observed before and after a total solar eclipse,
a multitude of faint ripples, a moving sourceless light,
refracting eddies through miles of atmosphere.
Each day now I'm eclipsed and abandoned

in a riptide of lightless shadows
across the sea where Mothra waits
on her island for her child to be born.

13   Center Piece

Stepping through wet grass,
we had to wait until this morning,
the morning of the service,
that is to happen early in the afternoon
so the cut flowers will be fresh,
not wilted for someone who is late
and no longer waiting to be later.
Stopping repeatedly on the shoulderless
gravel road to cut clusters of yellow coneflowers,
brown-eyed susans, rattlesnake grass,
lanky blue stem, flowering Indian grass,
and the blunt-brown silent towers of cattails
that will rise blind over the round
wooden tables at the reception.

From the pulpit, two people share stories of the man
who is late, a classic old-time fiddler
who at square dances and stage performances,
as he grew older, would keep playing
even after he'd fallen asleep.
When the song ended the banjo player
would brush against him so he'd open his eyes,
but not startled, completing the phrase.
It's the best any of us can hope for.

14 Friday at Volunteer Park

Beyond the radiated area, shower water runs down my back, leaving a wet raging fire, a soaking burn. The doctor informs me that a majority of radiation patients experience shingles regardless of receiving the shingles shot.

Mid-afternoon sleeves of light
blow loosely through evergreens.

An explosion of relaxation
spreads across the kept lawn.

Traffic beyond the well-groomed hedges
practices for its rush hour charge.

The splintered glass of dragonflies
glitters in and out of deep shadows.

A blond lab is eager to retrieve a tennis ball.
Frisbees rise, fall, are caught.

The initial-gouged picnic table leans downhill
with no message of reprieve for Jack and Jill.

Fir spires cathedral up in mythic
green rings, altar for blue sky.

Perhaps this explains all these work-wounded bodies
lying in the grass, exposing what they can

on their makeshift blanket stretchers,
soon to be folded and carried home to dinner.

Most surrender their reading, books left open
and face down. A tent bivouac of scattered

unfinished stories, mark the place where the day's
glory ended, even as the grass reads ahead.

This is what we volunteered to do
then are drafted to die in other ways.

15   Misdiagnosed Eclipse

After today's radiation swept my body back into my clothes, it's time for the weekly doctor visit. Walking the hall in chili-peppered socks, my back to the foot-thick lead-lined door, I turn right. Since shingles presents itself asymmetrically, something I learned last week, I'm concerned about the cluster of red blotches reaching up to my right armpit, more like bloody footprints on my skin. Am I guilty of attacking myself? Really, probably, a conquistador still in search of the Seven Cities of Cibola and leaving gifts of smallpox.

No, I'm told it's chigger bites from standing out in the middle of a back forty that was mowed to reduce a tick infestation. It didn't help me through the moon's total eclipse. Now I'm eclipsed by itching. I keep telling myself suffering is the price of worth. But that's not all, my right big toe is so painful that I'm limping and don't want to wear shoes. The nurse says the pain sounds like 8 on a 10-point scale. Well, I could just wear one shoe, but then I'd have a limp to beat the sheriff's sidekick Chester in that 50s TV western Gunsmoke. Since my right side is under attack, I wonder if this is related to the radiation. No, it's an attack of gout. This happens sometimes with patients. The technician asks if the doctor mentioned this. True or not, there's so much not told, hidden or lost somewhere in clouds of radiation.

∞

Our faces anonymous with sky.
Now we know what we watched as children
on summer afternoons was real, not fake news:
legions of sheep herded by doggéd winds,
invading armadas of three-masted ships
quickly sinking below the horizon,
all the animals that ran wild, freed from a broken-down
three-ringed circus, but it's too late to report it,
no one will believe us, the ones with our heads
bent back and faces erased by darkening sky.
Planets and a few stars unbound by day's bright chains.
A gold-ringed porthole appears where we fall
into emptiness where not even nothing exits.

∞

Heads bent back for at least an hour, maybe less,
our cervical vertebrae now many stone arches of many bridges,
each spanning a life. On the surface of creeks,
the voluptuous reflections of passing clouds.
One man claims he can't get them out of his eyes
even with his eyelids closed. Clouds tattooed deep
into the shimmer of his vitreous humor though someone
shouts out floaters as his eyes disintegrate into darkness.

∞

I search the gravel bar for a half-flat stone
then half bend my arm back to skip it
across the backwater pool where it skips across
the sky as the sky skips across the pool
and too quickly the stone is eclipsed
by water as the moon eclipses the sun.
A few stars briefly appear, the night insects
chorale a chorus then fall silent as the moon
skips onward out of the afternoon.

16   Any Week Now

The sign over the door, *Subwaiting Room.*
Though it has nothing to do with submersibles,
it has everything to do with being submerged .

Wednesday:
Have you seen your doctor today?
    No, I see him on Thursdays.
Oh, I see mine on Wednesdays
before chemo. Radiation the rest
of the week.

Thursday:
You know anything new?
    No, not really.
Well, the day ain't over with yet.
    Maybe something will come along.

Friday:
On Monday the doctor said I was stage one.
After the PET scan he said stage three.

This patient sailor logs a thousand miles a week
for a series of five different types
of chemotherapy dripped into his body.
It really knocked the pudding
out of me two days ago.
His head leans hard into the wall
behind his chair. He opens his eyes,
I need to cut the hay in my fields
but one of my tractors is down.
His blue and white striped gown half open.

This is not the Admiral Lounge in a distant airport:
refuge for frequent flyers, veterans,
business class, all sipping on their complimentary
beverages. The treatment staff is behind schedule.

We are not rising up, autumn geese off a lake,
rather we are digging into drought stricken
Midwestern dirt. Neither of us
wears a watch. We wear the age we are.
Time alludes and eludes us.

17   Populus Deltoides or Pinus Echinata?

Maybe it's a question that most of us are asked
in elementary school, or maybe not, but something
that most of wish we were asked at one time or another,
but then never answer to anyone's satisfaction,
including our own. Teacher and classmates smirk
and giggle at confessions of tree and bark,
sure that each of us is barking up the wrong tree.

We are left to the silence of wooden hallways,
then forget about answers and questions
and learn no matter how poorly
to place one root in front of the other,
walking or dragging the growing weight
of who we are and who we never
imagined being, and this time it is not
a question but a correction and a declaration.

I stand in the medical office,
underwear pulled down just enough
to follow the straight trail of reddish blotches
across my waist, wandering tracks of a lonely animal
over dunes of flesh, a desert searching for a lost body.
It's moved up the right side of my chest
to nest in my armpit and then down
the other side, but not an animal either
as the doctor declares pityriasis (Christmas Tree) rosea.

Yes, I'm a tree and I know it's true. I live in a tree house
surrounded by other trees, entangled, smothered by them,
unable to see farther than twenty feet through summer foliage.

I've walked up to the cottonwood on the north side
of the garden, hugged it with both arms and thanked
it for growing in such an unexpected place, so far
from others of its kind. I've fretted when it dropped
half of its leaves during droughts and watered it,

accidentally leaving the hydrant hose running for hours.
Its trunk now over two feet in diameter and fifty feet tall,
I'm such a small thing to hug something so large.

Now in late summer, I'm a Christmas tree
decorated with red ornaments, the cause unknown,
maybe a virus, a junk diagnosis according to the doctor.
Maybe it will go away in a month,
no one knows how deep the roots go
or how long the ornaments will hang
before falling and breaking into a different diagnosis.

18   Revelry

> Timothy Leary's dead.
> No, no, no, no, he's outside looking in.
> —Moody Blues

Laid out on the carbon-fiber table
waiting for the scintillating lasers and fission
to redress me, I stare at the drop ceiling panels.

One white panel replaced with a backlit multi-colored
transparency, a glowing window into rocky snow-capped
mountains where, in the foreground, a dirt trail ascends.

∞

There's a window on my tongue
panes of lemon juice, a tomato sunset, either way
I'm not climbing into mountains.

How many more times can this wallpaper die
before its wounds open wide enough
and begin to exuberantly peel?

Maybe a wrecking ball will open the wall
or a missile open the building
spilling its contents into the day's news.

Let in some light even on this overcast day
in a city whose allegiance is to the overcast.
Let in some air shadowed by a downtrodden rain.

∞

No matter what I say
or try not to say I see through. No need
for window washers on this floor.

The lower sash stays open for the fruit flies and wasps,
maybe birds and bees, to enter and leave without perching
on the sharp shards of existence.

Pricking the doubters and believers alike,
serving up the desperate hunger
of the terminally alive, knowing

that the universe is mostly based
upon belief whether it is true
Or not, even as the floor dissolves.

$$\infty$$

Actually, the window on the tip of my tongue
is framed by taste buds and not a mountain.
Windows taste like paper soaked in watermelon sugar.

Decades ago, at a surprise 40th birthday party,
a friend decided it was time to best himself,
to break out a city of window panes that was stored

in a repurposed mayonnaise jar in his refrigerator
to preserve and induce the freshest visions. He greeted each
arriving car at the entrance to the long gravel driveway,

where he administered a window pane to each adult
for their near and far trip to the future. When I returned
home from work my surprise was preoccupied

with the gathering chaos.
Sitting at the kitchen table,
I drank a cup of coffee,

tempted by a baseball-glove-sized pretzel
that was knotted into a salty heart
only to discover that I did have a window pane

on my tongue, gift from the cup,
a sly surprise, a present to the day
opening and reopening into evening,

opening into a frayed and holy world,
opening to the clear panes beyond and behind
everything that I might say and will ever say.

      ∞

The linear accelerator begins its work tracing three microdot
tattoos as I walk along the trail through bear grass
and Indian paintbrush deeper into the Cold Mountains.

19   Table Dates

The radiology technicians, the nurses, the doctors,
at one time or another, but always first thing each morning,
want to know my birthdate. As if the date were prone
to warping in a decaying half-life, to fission shifts of space/time,
to earthquake slippage, to being chin-deep in floods,
to be buried under landslides, or out bursts of irrational radiation,
and maybe that's all possible if shifting means forgetting
where all the pieces were left, not knowing what was lost,
jostled in the trunk of a beat-up Grand Am rushing down
some backroad looking for a place to dump the evidence.

Still it's annoying to keep repeating myself
as if I can no longer be trusted, wallowing in
desperation to escape or unable to stand up
to some moral failure that can't be acknowledged.
But it might be nice to be a few years younger
so I change the year but not the day and month.
No one notices a difference in two decades.
Asked if I could live my life over again
would I do anything different, as if I'm already
a beached castaway, or worse, written off—
the guarantee, the extended warranty
not worth the paper it's not printed on.

∞

If I can't think of something new,
but I know it's my fault, not just because I don't remember
my first breath even as I'm trying to breathlessly
backstroke away from my last one on this narrow table
in a too strong undertow that yanks me farther
out toward agitated horizons of failure,
where sea and sky dissolve into each other.
If I'm not flying with a flock of pelicans,
I'm swimming through a turbulent sea of electrons.

The big event that occurred on my new birth date,
that makes me younger by twenty years

was the first moon walk.
There are skeptics who believe it was staged
by Hollywood and the *gov'ment*.
One evangelical preacher's only interest
is to leave a Bible on the moon
just in case we blow ourselves up,
just in case some stranger shows up
who can read English.
I'm hanging ten on my back
on a table more narrow than a surf board
trying to stay afloat drenched in a downpouring fission.

20 Camaraderie

The day after Labor Day, standing in the produce
section of Clover's Health Food Store, talking
with a man whose prostatectomy was
a few years earlier than mine. Now his PSA is
creeping upward. Half-bent over the cooler, he's
shaking water from a small bundle of cilantro
before placing it in his cart. I'm over-eating free
sliced samples of diva apples. He says he likes
the piñata apples better. I've got two
and a half weeks more of mid-morning rendezvous
with the linear accelerator as it mounts me,
whispers to each side of my hips then swings
so its rays penetrate every fleshy fiber
of what I can't feel. He says that he may be following
in my footsteps, but I don't know the way,
and will have to wait at least nine months
before I know if there is another way,
that is oceans away. He wanders
to the other end of the produce aisle
to pick up an eggplant.

PSA: Prostate Specific Antigen

21   Sea Space in the Parking Lot

In the event that this is the ocean,
an ancient ocean, I follow the sidewalk
that follows the edge of a parking lot,
that slips down before gently rising back up,
a slow swelling tide of concrete or a blue whale
surfacing in the swales as a tidal wind fingers
my hair, sweeping in a gray mist to veil
the known world that I'm losing
as I inhale the salty Midwestern air.

A beach covered with the greenest grass.
After a century, these crowning oaks rise
out of the waves and shake themselves dry,
dog-like, a loose leafy pack out for the day,
chasing sun-loving seals that bark back
and lumber toward the constant churning grass.
The mongrels always busy, distracted, reclassifying
what's left of the dead and almost dead,
including the intact but empty red crab shell the size
of a baseball glove left permanently catching barnacles.

A single engine piper cub flies past, parallel
to the towel-bound, sun-loving crowd, not far out
over the green mown water, as it trails a long sign,
NOW IS THE TIME, as if the sky had any other choice,
is the bluest Hershey's Kiss about to be opened,
if only I could pull the little paper tab hard enough,
a ripcord, and then parachute into that gleaming
hallway of darkness and not just this daily dying.

22 Revolution Number Nine

It's all too much to assume but who cares,
anyone who lived through the 60s and 70s decades
and may now still want a revolution.

I walk out the double glass doors
into sunlight that has the clarity
of having been touched too deeply,
declaring every blade of grass a relative of Whitman
with Blake waiting for each sand grain
to be hurled into new worlds.

I see only barricades of light that need
to be mounted, shot through with waves,
with particles, throngs of space unfurling
thonged banners and feckless flags,
all hand-sewn from rags.
An army of mimes gesture
for the many crowds of one walking by
on the sidewalk to join and break open
the day's Bastille doors, to free
the prisoners to build their own guillotines
and decapitate their diagnoses.

∞

Back in the subwaiting room
the conspirators continue to plot:

*I'm just blown away at how many people
are walking through here.*

*My white blood cell count is low
so I couldn't do chemo and radiation today.
I'll miss out on getting wacked twice.*

So many *bless yous* and *God be with you*
and then the room is quiet until the new man
wonders why there isn't a shot that would

resolve all this as the conversation turns
to where they once were, then left,
and now return, before good or bad, it is all
to be forgotten: the little town whose name was . . .
and no one can recall . . . but there was a moment,
the one at the Ford dealership, maybe east on 36
leaving highway 63 behind, the cabala of work,
not Kirksville, Green Top, Queen City,
but Lancaster or Unionville, where the job
was delivering washed, folded uniforms
and shop towels, when one day the young
driver hid a rubber snake in a pile of laundry
and the old man who sorted the clothes,
who was deathly afraid of snakes,
nearly died of a heart attack,
as all revolutions of the living
die in the dirty details.

23   Treading Time

Our watches break, too cheap
to be anything but throwaways.

Batteries fail, the small hands frozen
at 9 and 3 as if falling open armed into a wet day.

Time stretched into a dead-man's float,
suspended under a glass crystal.

Such a pathetic gesture: the infinite organized, the eternal
regimented, eventually marched off to another endless war.

Time's shotgun wedding with space, their novaed honeymoon
scattered across the universe. No divorce court here.

Maybe a half-life sucked soon enough
into a parallel dimension,

With a digital watch I don't have to envision,
flailing hands and arms frantically waving for a rescue,

Assured I will never arrive. Nothing good to come of it.
chairs in the subwaiting room so uncomfortable.

24   Seven Miscalculations

Too unpredictable, these seven circles of hell,
even when there are nine.
And seven steps to heaven?
Why not six, eight, eleven?
Twelve steps to a shaky sobriety.
Twelve to walk up to the second floor
of this house and eleven down,
one for a defenestration and media notoriety.
Over twenty to reach the office
on the second floor where I worked
for twenty years and almost never returned.

Who's counting?
Do we hope the sums to be aerobically lavish?
Hope's hope for a greater sum than the parts?
Add in a few more steps,
a hop, skip, a long jump,
that wins a bronze medal,
and a few years later, retirement
a long jump with torn ligaments.

Double the chances, the Seven-Eleven quick-stop
on the corner of Hitt and Locust.
A collision of collusions.
Future plagues cast into the dumpster.
The midnight flash flood of the homeless
holding sixty-four ounce slurpees,
inundating the dark alleys and begging for more.

Accept, acquiesce, attenuate the attention,
maybe, finally, ultimately, a healing
but not a cure. We at the calendar's
short end, resigned to a life, the lack of it,
the end closer for the near-sighted.

Complexity to congest insight
to distract the terminally alive—
a leap beyond tragedy into statistics—
the piss-stained pole over the curb
from where the streetlight flickers,
a mechanical candle in night's collapsing dome.
To see what is in sight, seven parked cars,
seven upturned cups overflowing
from their executioners, then to see
beyond our sightless seeing.

25   RSVP/RIP

What's charred is charred. The weekend to recover.
A couple we see every two or three years,
invites us to dinner. By the time we leave,
much later than planned, and after too much
of everything including laughter and hysterical stories
of grandkids gone awry, hateful daughters-in-law,
a son's divorce and his other son's new girlfriend
that they swear to keep around even if their son doesn't,
and then the drive to his older sister's house
who has taken in two indigent young men,
foisted on her by her only son who steals
her money and sells most everything of value
in the house until she has nothing left.
   ∞

He didn't holster either of the two illegal hand guns
taken from his brother who only had suicide
in mind. He did throw a baseball bat
on the front seat of his pickup just in case.
He's screaming in my face, his wrinkles
a twisting topography of a past war that knows
no past as he rushes to describe how he threatened
everyone in his sister's house,
telling one young man dressed in coat and tie,
getting ready for a job interview,
that every time he flushes the toilet
he's costing his sister money.
   ∞

Across the table, he drinks another beer
and says it was in his first fire fight
in 'Nam, amid the insane gun fire,
the blinding, deafening explosions, the teenager
huddled next to him slumped over curling
into a fetal position. Screaming for the corpsman,
who dove in behind the sandbags
and into the trench with them, who lifted

the upper lip of the man that he was cradling
in his arms, and across the dinner table where he now sits
his own arms folded across his body as if rocking a baby.
There was a perfectly round bullet hole, AK-47,
between the soldier's two front teeth. The corpsman
bent the man's head forward to find the exit wound
in the back of his neck, there was a fist-sized hole.
Putting down his empty beer can, he says, he threw
the whimpering soldier over his shoulder and carried him
through the cover of jungle to a medevac chopper.
He always wonders if the wounded man survived.
He sees his face often in the grocery store and corner bar.

Diagnosed: Agent Orange-induced prostate cancer,
he's been cancer free for eighteen years.
I made it one and a half years
before beginning radiation. We both know,
nothing is ever settled.

26   Sunday

Across the yard into the woods
that disappear down the hill into the creek,
under the leaf litter piled in the gutters,
in the back of the refrigerator that cries out
to be cleaned, the decomposing continues,
but no one is looking for the outcome,
just another day of waiting for news
and a few more chance encounters.

27   Six Left

Only the first digit of the beast.
Mathematics the language of heaven
if you're a mathematician.

The beast howling in his bed
and the number pushing a friend
to call me to his hospital room.

His speech always hesitant, doubtful,
apprehensive, as if falling from his mouth
and not spoken, all he could not speak.

This day he'd make John Wayne
sound loquacious. I visit him
on the sixth floor of the north hospital tower,

knowing I'm down to six more treatments,
six mornings of the red laser beam
tracking my escape.

He's now a stroke patient.
It was proceeded by a series of unnoticed
mini-strokes before he collapsed

on his porch that overlooks a dry creek bed
late this summer. He couldn't walk.
The ambulance struggled to make the turn,

dragging its rear bumper up the rocky bank.
No medical directive, no will.
No time for second thoughts.

Third ones belong to the other side
of the universe. I'm sure that he can't
hear this. The prey can't stop running.

The hunter and the hunted
caught out of breath
in the same stumbling stride.

28   Ultima Thule

This is the day I forget to forget
that this day will never
be so carefree and careless again.

A cold stone tossed coldly
into the pond. I huddle close to shore.
The stalk of every cattail shivers,
small angular dirt clods tumble down the bank,
into the water, smaller waves ricochet, cross
and recross themselves, diminished penitents
returning to their center where I will last as long
as I tread water as if practicing for a shipwreck .

Half life? Half alive? Halfway and one step
more. Halfway back not the way.
Then much less than half even as the rising
of autumn's harvest moon aims its full barrel
of light at the field embalmed in a photo
on the kitchen calendar.

The linear accelerator whirs around me,
dives at the narrow table and forces me
to lie still. Now I'm told it's called stereotactic body
radiation therapy. It's all in a name. Conan
where are you, defend me from this barbarian?

Two hip and one pubic tattoo centered
below my navel keep the beams aligned
as it burns away rampantly dividing cells
that are busy burying me.

29   Little League

Was it extending my tongue to lick
one too many envelopes: electric,
water, gas, phone bills, the regular dose
of glue month after month for decades?

Was it grinding a lifetime of coffee,
each morning the whirling electric motor
radiating a counter-high electromagnetic field
as I leaned in to smell the rich aroma?

Was it that I didn't start drinking coffee
until I was 29, needing
something to keep me moving
through the diesel fumes, dodging
bulldozers, backhoes, and toppling cranes?

Was it the strontium-90, cesium-137, iodine-131,
Americium-241, drifting across the 1950s A-bomb-tested
continent, drifting over our young bodies, turning us into
down-winders, as they did their best to destroy us,
calling it safety, defense, security?

Was it the chlorine, fluoride, hormones,
teflon, aluminum pots, micro-plastics swirling
in every glass and swimming pool that flowed
over and through us each summer,
then reduced to endless acronyms: DDT, BPA?

Was it knocking over salt shakers one
too many times and forgetting to throw
a pinch over a left or right shoulder,
confusing which side is more effective
at avoiding collateral damage?

Was it the mismatched socks
that were a growing imbalance,

a stumbling stride, heading
in too many directions
for my mutating molecules?

Was it living too close to
high voltage electric lines
and Roundup sprayed along
their meandering across creeks
and down into valleys?

Was it the fungus a friend claims
is the root of all bodily evil?
Was it sticking my head out
the back seat window of a '58

green Oldsmobile to inhale
the sweet petroleum fumes
in the gas station on our way
to little league baseball games?

30   Row, Row, Row Your Dream

∞

No light enters or leaves through these four walls—
submerged in the subwaiting room.
No smell of sea air or diesel, only the gurgle
of water in the fountain outside the door.
There could be a tide in the cooler
but not deep enough to float
a rowboat to escape the cartoon sinking.

A periscope descends from the ceiling.
No one reaches for it, waiting
for the captain to issue orders.
Patients stare at four pastel horizons
where smoke rises from distant torpedoed ships,
their bows point down into a tranquil sea
as small oil-slicked stick figures
jump over the flaming railings.

∞

Cruising the middle of a river
as if this were still Saturday
and heroes still possible,
five women and three men in
a canopied pontoon boat.
No one notices the small wake
cut by the periscope
that follows them toward the Gulf
a thousand miles of river current south.
No epic intentions to guide them
except to get through the day.
Empty beer bottles rattle, fall, clang
against the boat's gunwale and into the hull.

A drunken syrupy panic fills the boat,
no one sure what their roles are
except to die. A siren's crucifying wail

and the pontoon boat drops depth charges.
In the first flush of explosions,
the boat is surrounded by the floating
bodies of twenty-pound Asian carp.
Nuclear torpedoes fired, miss their target,
bury themselves in the steep mud
of the riverbank to await a future Fourth of July.

∞

We sit quietly in the subwaiting
room with cartoon versions
of ourselves. Why not believe it all.
We can't get any of it back anyway.
I spin the periscope back around,
we are the ruins of our childhoods.

31   The Sea Shall Free Us

Pants left hanging in the locker, I pull
from the clean bleached stack on the bench
a folded gown. Arms raised
above my head, I am the sailor from
a one-man defeated navy.
I slip into the sleeves and the sea's gown flutters
down my exposed back. The fog does not part
to my passing. Each day gravity dresses me
in finely striped blue and white linen,
without hope of floating above the waiting line
of other gowned ghosts wondering
when their ships will return to a safe harbor.

The disembodied voice over the intercom
too clear but not enough to clear anything up
except another man disappears in the depths of the hall.
If there is time to say what I have not said before,
I only discover that I am struck dumb amongst
the waiting where no one listens as the fathoms
of wet silence pressurize the deep.

It's not a gown but a life jacket.
Each of us holds our breath and tries
to reach a surface that is breathable.
A few of us know to dive deeper
where we stare into each other's eyes
before we drown into another day.

32 Decompression

There is so little time to think
that there is so little time.
Dust swirls between words,
sentences, raw syllables,
that haven't been spoken in eons.
Archeologists excavate each other
and discover that they aren't all
that interesting until they don grim
golden masks intimating what by now
they should know better, even as the journals
reject their articles on the emergence
of amphora with rounded lips found
neatly stacked in the rotting hull
of another Roman shipwreck, and the monographs
on the domestication of wind,
the harnessing of spoons, ad infinitum of the fantastic,
that takes up the little time that's left
except for the time being, being in time
in the subwaiting room.

33   Caught in the Undertow

It's a healing not a cure.
It's a hole but maybe a window.
It's a passageway blocked by scars,
guarded by a sentinel who claims
no one passes without his approval,
and, of course, a bribe, and being young,
at least youthful, will get you up
the gang plank for the cruise.

The stethoscope moon swings
from his neck even on cloudy days.
He's rated as an expert marksman
with a slingshot of radioactive isotope.
Even with poor visibility
and listening posts in no-man's land
defense is a sham, my end always in sight
even if I refuse to watch, departing Strand's Harbor.

No matter how quickly I unmake myself,
turning away clinging to whatever jacket
I cherish, rabbit's foot and worry stone
in each hand, remembering the instructions
are to pull the red tab to inflate
before jumping into the turbulent waves
of another hour, praying the radio operator
is able to send one more SOS
before the currents wash me far out to sea.

34   Four Minutes and Thirty-Three Seconds

Staccato laughter from a door down the hall
on the way to the linear accelerator.
A cackle rises from around the cauldron
of a desktop computer.
A new man comes back from treatment
who knows this is my last day.
I think that every day.
We awkwardly shake hands like rubbing
two sticks together hoping to kindle a fire
without smoke, and we wish each other
the best. Always the best.

He's just happy to have this day.
He's at the beginning of his radiation
therapy. He just wants more time to keep moving.
I don't ask where. *Doing the best I can,* he says,
and can't stop smiling. Outside the subwaiting room,
a patient is being advised to check with the financial
department to see if there is a fund for gas money.
A passing nurse says he should have done that
at the beginning of treatment. The man says he's just
looking for gas money for the follow up care.
It's too easy to say we are all running on empty
whether we are smiling or not.

Maybe it's better to be standing on the side
of the road, thumb out in the direction
he thinks he's headed. To the horizon,
not a car in sight in either lane, only a breeze
rustling dry weeds and a grasshopper clicking
away in harmony with John Cage,
when a nuclear submarine's periscope
cuts the black asphalt surface like a scalpel,
pulls up on the gravel shoulder and stops,
its deck hatch open and waiting.

35   Washed Up

The coast crying out for tragedy like all beautiful places.
                                                —Robinson Jeffers

After the hammer crash of the churning crest,
What's left of the wave thrashes on the shore
As if some shy, fearful thing from the deep-submerged,
Shocked by the salt-stormed air, wants back under.

The wave draws down and rounded pebbles
Follow its ebbing leash amid bone rattle
And shell clatter, leaving the polished wet granite
And broken glass dulled above the tide's reach.

Against hard tidal winds, sand hisses
Racing for the lee of what's left standing
And lying down, not yet buried, their grainy shadows
Reaching beyond the wave-toss and loss.

The beach with high tide's edges posted.
The rusted signs of lonely warnings that go unheeded,
Unable to turn back the sea's dissolving into sky,
And loosening the horizon, read:

>   *Beach Logs Kill* and all around
>   in the pattern of pick-up-sticks shoved aside
>   for another gamey day, is chain-sawed timber
>   the diameter of garage doors, the length of jets.
>
>   *Beware of Mountain Lion Attacks*
>   with little to be done but stroll a hungry universe,
>   barefoot between dislodged barnacles, scuttling crabs,
>   and the cry of swooping gulls feeding along the shimmer.
>
>   *Ocean Makes the Rules*,
>   As if it'd been forgotten that *Eternity is not measured
>   in duration*, I wade ankle deep
>   in the salt spray sweeping the infinite shore.

36 Return to the Sea

And the astonished children, not knowing
where they came from and soon not caring,
only the day's chase down the beach
reminds them of how much farther they must go.

Surrounded by chaotic gulls, their comma splices
marking the sky's vast run-on sentence, the opening
and closing apostrophes of their wings, the unhinged
mewling, and the children with their own breaking

cries as the tide ebbs, pulls back with the worn out
until the wearing down leaves both of them translucent,
and the wind excites sand sweeping grains
of older worlds into finer shadows.

37   Ashes

Since I no longer have a prostate,
Eight out of twelve biopsy samples dense
With cancer, and during the prostatectomy,
It was discovered that the cancer
Had broken out of the prostate's seal,
And begun to spread up the right seminal vesicle.
So what's left is to radiate the prostate bed.
The linear accelerator, a mere 10 million
Dollar machine that spins electrons
At high rates of speed and then fires them
Through leaves of tungsten guided by lasers aligned
To pencil point hip tattoos that send radiation
Deep into my body setting cells on fire.

There are no fire trucks, no sirens screaming
To get out the way at the intersection
Of each morning, no lights manically flashing
Warnings, except for the lasers' glittering red lights
Parading across my lower torso, no leaking hoses
Tangling across the tile floor or hook and ladders
Raised to rescue my beleaguered body from the bottom
Floor of heaven. I lie back, let the fire spread,
And don't feel a thing. I must be dead already.
Months later, after a colonoscopy, the radiologist
Insists on a digital examine. My sex life for the year.

38   At Five in the Afternoon

In the shower
He took my towel.
He said I didn't need it anymore.
I stood there leaving puddles on the floor
As he whip-snapped it against my right buttock.

At five in the afternoon,
He took my shampoo and shower gel
Using the same lame excuse.
He said don't worry about
The broken toilet either. He'll call
A plumber whose last day
On the job is tomorrow.

What about my clothes,
My shirt and pants?
I can't get dressed wet.
He said don't worry about it.
Naked is de rigueur.
Everyone is naked with or without clothes.

What about driving my car naked?
No one will care, no one will see you,
Ever again. It will all be a figment
Of your imagination when you open
The door and step into where
You have never been before

Where you will never be again.
We have it all wrong,
The door is always open and closed,
Death is a burden and comfort,
It's the catacombs that stay in motion.

~ End Over End ~

39   Body Heist

His pudgy skin bloated from whatever drug regime and radiation is toppling his body toward a transcendent junta of worms. The bed elevated at a thirty-degree angle makes him chatty. He gesticulates emphatically on ancient ethical ephemera. From his quaquaversal Calvary of sheets and blankets, he's an avatar of wrong turns and dark alleys, of too slow beginnings and too quick ends, of missed opportunities and opportunities to miss.

His daughter, who lives with her mother, stopped by earlier. Not out of high school and she already has her first DUI, driving under the influence, his influence. His daughter is an accident in progress, moving to Atlanta, planting herself in an away world of expensive chariots and highways lined with billboards advertising new crosses to bear. Sideswiped, sidetracked, broadsided, side-showed, pain pikes his right hip, cancer latticed though his skeleton, tumors freshly burned and burning, a smoldering barbaric-bone-barbequed citadel, a body surrendering to a holy siege.

40   Why Twenty-Two Equals Thirty-Eight Divided by Seven

I passed through 38 and in long ago years,
but then I mostly didn't notice, or bother to count
that high or look that low, and it's mostly not a milestone,
maybe a passing mile marker along the interstate.
Yes, I missed the speedometer zip passed 38,
unacknowledged, too busy watching the road,
watching the merging traffic, watching it all pass so quickly,
reading the billboards, "Have your vasectomy reversed
in Florida," and "I make 10,000 mistakes then succeed."

The wide gray tongues of exit ramps lead
to the glare of gas stations, and don't bother
with the thought that 38 is far behind,
the dull black .38 Special dropped in some 1938 noir
murder mystery. The radio is tuned to an easy rock station
where I hear the band .38 Special fire off a blistering
guitar solo, and my destiny becomes a few chords
and fragments of lyrics that begin to repeat themselves
38 times in my head as my fingers tap out the next tune played,
"Running on Empty," there on top of the steering wheel
as I become attuned to the presence
of the past that is speeding to catch up and pass
someone who is wading through the number 38.

38 has been with us for longer than anyone
can remember: the year XXXVIII started on
a Wednesday of the Julian calendar, (in use today
only on Faulal, the most far flung island of the Shetlands),
known as the year of the Consulship of Julianus and Asprenas.
Has anyone asked those delinquent kids, Romulus and Remus,
about this or did a wolf's math education eat them up?
Did they know that 38 is the sum of the squares
of the first three prime numbers, that 38 is the largest
even number that can't be written as the sum of two odd
composite numbers, and with a little origami math
folding the first 8 of 88 vertically in half gives you 38.

Yes, 38 is everywhere, but Douglas Adams hitchhiking
across a parallel universe tells us that 42 is the answer
to all fundamental questions, yet decades ago,
driving the slopes of the Gila Mountains in New Mexico,
on a hairpin turn, a man came to a stop on an outside shoulder
beside a deep canyon with no guard rail. He was staring
into the silent roar of a silver sliver that was a river far below,
and then staring into the uproar of a blue desert sky,
beside his rusting Ford licensed with the mystical number
to the third power 22 22 22. The rusting Ford Galaxy's
windshield modified to hold 22 separate panes of glass.
He was giving away 22-dollar bills printed with his profile
in the center oval. He'd officially changed his name
to Love Twenty-Two. He siphoned gas from a van
using his mouth and a short section of hose
that he carried as if he'd done this many times before,
so he could make it to the next promised land,
but inadvertently swallowing too much of this combustible elixir,
he spent the afternoon retching. He hadn't yet risen to
the transcendence of ingested liquid hydrocarbons
as he declared himself forever to be 22 years old.
He brushed aside his gray hair and heaved once more
but not over the rock ledge where the gravity of fundamental
questions were left desiccated in the hot sun.

Omniscient, omnipotent 38:
the area code in the defunct country of Yugoslavia,
where phones still ring that no one answers,
38 the atomic number of the element strontium,
still uplifted in post-nuclear-testing of Southwest dust-storms,
38 the number exemplifying bravery in Norse myths
and some of us still bow before Valhalla's tree of life.
Still we wait a turn to spin the roulette wheel
with its 38 slots, waiting to share all the winners' winnings.
Casino workers working 38 years of tragic magic
still without health insurance and pensions.

It's only 7 steps to heaven according to the local 9th
and Broadway evangelist who stands in beat-down cowboy boots
on a green bus bench, conducting quitting time traffic,
his shouldered boombox blasting full volume as the long line
of brake lights trail off following like lasers working
over the swelling belly of an asphalt sea of darkness
counting backwards from 42 to 38 to 22.

OTHER BOOKS OF POETRY BY LAMAR UNIVERSITY LITERARY PRESS

Academy of Dreams Glover Davis
The Angled Road Jonas Zdanys
Betrayal Creek Kip Stratton
Black Sunday Benjamin Myers
The Bluebonnet Sutras Jerry Bradley
Collapsing into Possibility Jerry Bradley
Dear Dreamland Markham Johnson
The Family Book of Martyrs Benjamin Myers
First Light Lynn Hoggard
For Every Tatter Christine H. Boldt
Hamlet in Exile Ulf Kirchdorfer
Hungry Ghost Diner Kelly Ellis
A Lifetime of Words Jan Seale
Last Red Dirt Embrace W. K. Stratton
Ode to My Mother's Voice Loretta Diane Walker
Only So Many Autumns Betsy Joseph
Particulars Jan Seale
A Place Comfortable with Fire John Milkereit
A Room for Us Devan Burton
Relatively Speaking Chip Dameron and Betsy Joseph
Sailing West Carol Coffee Reposa
Some Electric Hum Janice Northerns
Some Vegetable Sacrifice Scott Yarbrough
Sports Page Ken Waldman
Yet at the Gates, a Refuge of Sunflowers and Milkweed Dan Williams

For more information, go to www.lamar.edu/literarypress

www.ingramcontent.com/pod-product-compliance
Lightning Source LLC
Chambersburg PA
CBHW071238090426
42736CB00014B/3130